KETO VEGETARIAN

MAIN COURSE RECIPES

Quick, Easy and Delicious Low Carb Recipes
for healthy living while keeping
your weight under control

Lisa Jackson

Copyright © 2021 by Lisa Jackson

Legal Disclaimer

The information contained in this book and its contents is not designed to replace any form of medical or professional advice; and is not meant to replace the need for independent medical, financial, legal, or other professional advice or service that may require. The content and information in this book have been provided for educational and entertainment purposes only.

The content and information contained in this book have been compiled from sources deemed reliable, and they are accurate to the best of the Author's knowledge, information and belief.

However, the Author cannot guarantee its accuracy and validity and therefore cannot be held liable for any errors and/or omissions.

Further, changes are periodically made to this book as needed. Where appropriate and/or necessary, you must consult a professional (including but not limited to your doctor, attorney, financial advisor, or other such professional) before using any of the suggested remedies, techniques, and/or information in this book.

Upon using this book's contents and information, you agree to hold harmless the Author from any damaged, costs and expenses, including any legal fees potentially resulting from the application of any of the information in this book. This disclaimer applies to any loss, damages, or injury caused by the use and application of this book's content, whether directly and indirectly, whether for breach of contract, tort, negligence, personal injury, criminal intent, or under any other circumstances.

You agree to accept all risks of using the information presented in this book. You agree that by continuing to read this book, where appropriate and/or necessary, you shall consult a professional (including but not limited to your doctor, attorney, financial advisor, or other such professional) before remedies, techniques, and/or information in this book.

TABLE OF CONTENTS

Cheesy Macaroni with Broccoli

Prep Time:10 minutes

Cook Time:25 minutes

Servings: 6

Ingredients

- ➢ 1/3 cup melted coconut oil
- ➢ ¼ cup nutritional yeast
- ➢ 1 tablespoon tomato paste
- ➢ 1 tablespoon dried mustard
- ➢ 2 garlic cloves, minced
- ➢ 1 ½ teaspoons salt
- ➢ ½ teaspoon ground turmeric
- ➢ 4 ½ cups almond milk
- ➢ 3 cups cauliflower florets, chopped
- ➢ 1 cup raw cashews, chopped
- ➢ 1 lb. shell pasta
- ➢ 1 tablespoon white vinegar
- ➢ 3 cups broccoli florets

Directions:

1. Place a suitably-sized saucepan over medium heat and add coconut oil.
2. Stir in mustard, yeast, garlic, salt, tomato paste, and turmeric.

3. Cook for 1 minute then add almond milk, cashews, and cauliflower florets.

4. Continue cooking for 20 minutes on a simmer.

5. Transfer the cauliflower mixture to a blender jug then blend until smooth.

6. Stir in vinegar and blend until creamy.

7. Fill a suitably-sized pot with salted water and bring it to a boil on high heat.

8. Add pasta to the boiling water.

9. Place a steamer basket over the boiling water and add broccoli to the basket.

10.   Cook until the pasta is al dente. Drain and rinse the pasta and transfer the broccoli to a bowl.

11.   Add the cooked pasta to the cauliflower-cashews sauce.

12.   Toss in broccoli florets, salt, and black pepper.

13.   Mix well then serve.

Nutrition: Calories: 40; Fat: 2.0g Protein: 5g Carbohydrates: 7g Fiber: 4g Sugar: 3g Sodium: 18mg

Chili Fennel

Prep Time:10 minutes

Cook Time:8 minutes

Servings: 4

Ingredients:

➢ 2 fennel bulbs, cut into quarters

➢ 3 tablespoons olive oil

➢ Salt and black pepper to the taste

➢ 1 garlic clove, minced

➢ 1 red chili pepper, chopped

➢ ¾ cup veggie stock

➢ Juice of ½ lemon

Directions:

1. Heat a pan that fits your Air Fryer with the oil over medium-high heat, add garlic and chili pepper, stir and cook for 2 minutes.

2. Add fennel, salt, pepper, stock, and lemon juice, toss to coat, introduce in your Air Fryer and cook at 350 ° F for at least 6 minutes.

3. Divide into plates and serve as a side dish.

Nutrition: Calories: 158 kcal Protein: 3.57 g Fat: 11.94 g Carbohydrates: 11.33 g

Collard Greens and Tomatoes

Prep Time:10 minutes

Cook Time:10 minutes

Servings: 9

Ingredients:

- ➢ 1 pound collard greens
- ➢ ¼ cup cherry tomatoes, halved
- ➢ 1 tablespoon apple cider vinegar
- ➢ 2 tablespoons veggie stock
- ➢ Salt and black pepper to the taste

Directions:

1. In a pan that fits the Air Fryer, combine tomatoes, collard greens, vinegar, stock, salt, and pepper, stir, introduce in your Air Fryer and cook at 320 ° F for 10 minutes.
2. Divide between plates and serve as a side dish.

Nutrition: Calories: 28 kcal Protein: 2.34 g Fat: 0.99 g Carbohydrates: 3.26 g

Bean and Carrot Spirals

Prep Time:10 minutes

Cook Time:40 minutes

Servings: 24

Ingredients:

- ➢ 4 8-inch flour tortillas
- ➢ 1 ½ cups of Easy Mean White Bean dip
- ➢ 10 ounces spinach leaves
- ➢ ½ cup diced carrots
- ➢ ½ cup diced red peppers

Directions:

1. Starts by preparing the bean dip, seen above. Next, spread out the bean dip on each tortilla, making sure to leave about a ¾ inch white border on the tortillas' surface. Next, place spinach in the center of the tortilla, followed by carrots and red peppers.

2. Roll the tortillas into tight rolls, and cover every rolls with plastic wrap or aluminum foil.

3. Let them chill in the fridge for twenty-four hours.

4. Afterward, remove the wrap from the spirals and remove the very ends of the rolls. Slice the rolls

into six individual spiral pieces, and arrange them on a platter for serving. Enjoy!

Nutrition: Calories: 205 kcal Protein: 6.41 g Fat: 4.16 g Carbohydrates: 35.13 g

Tofu Nuggets with Barbecue Glaze

Prep Time:10 minutes

Cook Time:25 minutes

Servings: 9

Ingredients:

➢ 32 ounces tofu

➢ 1 cup quick vegan barbecue sauce

Directions:

1. Set the oven to 425F.
2. Next, slice the tofu and blot the tofu with clean towels. Next, slice and dice the tofu and completely eliminate the water from the tofu material.
3. Stir the tofu with the vegan barbecue sauce, and place the tofu on a baking sheet.
4. Bake the tofu for fifteen minutes. Afterward, stir the tofu and bake the tofu for an additional ten minutes.
5. Enjoy!

Nutrition: Calories: 311 kcal Protein: 19.94 g Fat: 21.02 g Carbohydrates: 15.55 g

Vegetable and Chickpea Loaf

Prep Time:10 minutes

Cook Time:15 minutes

Servings: 4

Ingredients:

- 1 tsp. Salt
- .5 tsp. Dried sage
- 1 tsp. Dried savory
- 1 tbsp. Soy sauce
- .25 cup Parsley
- .5 cup Breadcrumbs
- .75 cup Oats
- .75 cup Chickpea flour
- 1.5 cup cooked chickpeas
- 2 Minced garlic cloves
- 1 Chopped yellow onion
- 1 Shredded carrot
- 1 Shredded white potato

Directions:

1. Set the oven to 350F. Take out a loaf pan and then grease it up.

2. Squeeze out the liquid from the potato and add to the food processor with the garlic, onion, and carrot.
3. Add the chickpeas and pulse to blend well. Add in the rest of the ingredients here, and when it is done, use your hands to form this into a loaf and add to the pan.
4. Place into the oven to bake for a bit until it is nice and firm. Let it cool down and then slice.

Nutrition: Calories: 351 kcal Protein: 16.86 g Fat: 6.51 g Carbohydrates: 64 g

Thyme and Lemon Couscous

Prep Time:5 minutes

Cook Time:10 minutes

Servings: 6

Ingredients:

- ➢ .25 cup Chopped parsley
- ➢ 1.5 cup Couscous
- ➢ 2 tbsp. Chopped thyme
- ➢ Juice and zest of a lemon
- ➢ 2.75 cup Vegetable stock

Directions:

1. Take out a pot and add in the thyme, lemon juice, and vegetable stock. Stir in the couscous after it has gotten to a boil and then take off the heat.

2. Allow sitting covered until it can take in all of the liquid. Then fluff up with a form.

3. Stir in the parsley and lemon zest, then serve warm.

Nutrition: Calories: 922 kcal Protein: 2.7 g Fat: 101.04 g Carbohydrates: 10.02 g

Baked Okra and Tomato

Prep Time:10 minutes

Cook Time:75 minutes

Servings: 6

Ingredients:

- ½ cup lima beans, frozen
- 4 tomatoes, chopped
- 8 ounces okra, fresh and washed, stemmed, sliced into ½ inch thick slices
- 1 onion, sliced into rings
- ½ sweet pepper, seeded and sliced thin
- Pinch of crushed red pepper
- Salt to taste

Directions:

1. Preheat your oven to 350 degrees Fahrenheit
2. Cook lima beans in water accordingly and drain them, take a 2quart casserole tin
3. Add all listed ingredients to the dish and cover with foil, bake for 45 minutes
4. Uncover the dish, stir well and bake for 35 minutes more
5. Stir then serve, and enjoy!

Nutrition: Calories: 55 Fat: 0g Carbohydrates: 12g Protein: 3g

Curried Apple

Prep Time:10 minutes

Cook Time:90 minutes

Servings: 4

Ingredients:

- ➢ 1 tablespoon fresh lemon juice
- ➢ ½ cup of water
- ➢ 2 apples, Fuji or Honeycrisp, cored and thinly sliced into rings
- ➢ 1 teaspoon curry powder

Directions:

1. Set the oven to 200F, take a rimmed baking sheet and line with parchment paper
2. Take a bowl and mix in lemon juice and water, add apples and soak for 2 minutes
3. Pat them dry and arrange in a single layer on your baking sheet, dust curry powder on top of apple slices
4. Bake for 45 minutes. After 45 minutes, turn the apples and bake for 45 minutes more
5. Let them cool for extra crispiness, serve and enjoy!

Nutrition: Calories: 240 Fat: 13g Carbohydrates: 20g Protein: 6g

Wild Rice and Millet Croquettes

Prep Time:5 minutes

Cook Time:20 minutes

Servings: 4

Ingredients:

- ¾ cooked millet
- ½ cup cooked wild rice
- 3 tablespoons extra virgin olive oil
- ¼ cup onion, minced
- 1 celery rib, finely minced
- ¼ cup carrot, shredded
- 1/3 cup all-purpose flour
- ¼ cup fresh parsley, chopped
- 2 teaspoons dried dill weed
- Salt and pepper to taste

Directions:

1. Add cooked millet and wild rice to a large-sized bowl, keep it to one side
2. Take a medium skillet and add 1 tablespoon of oil, place it over medium heat
3. Put onion, celery, and carrot and cook for at least 5 minutes

4. Add veggies and stir in flour, parsley, salt, pepper, and dill weed

5. Mix well and transfer to the fridge, let it sit for 20 minutes

6. Use hands to shape mixture into small patties, take a large skillet and place it over medium heat

7. Add 2 tablespoons of oil and let it heat up

8. Add croquettes and cook for 8 minutes in total until golden brown

9. Serve and enjoy!

Nutrition: Calories: 250 Fat: 9g Carbohydrates: 33g Protein: 9g

Grilled Eggplant Steaks

Prep Time:10 minutes

Cook Time:10 minutes

Servings: 4

Ingredients:

- ➢ 4 Roma tomatoes, diced
- ➢ 8 ounces cashew cream
- ➢ 2 eggplants
- ➢ 1 tablespoon olive oil
- ➢ 1 cup parsley, chopped
- ➢ 1 cucumber, diced
- ➢ Salt and pepper to taste

Directions:

1. Slice eggplants into three thick steaks, drizzle with oil, and season with salt and pepper
2. Grill in a pan for 4 minutes per side
3. Top with remaining ingredients
4. Serve and enjoy!

Nutrition: Calories: 86 Fat: 7g Carbohydrates: 12g Protein: 8g

Steamed Cauliflower

Prep Time: 5 minutes

Cook Time: 10 minutes

Servings: 6

Ingredients:

- ➤ 1 large head cauliflower
- ➤ 1 cup water
- ➤ ½ teaspoon salt
- ➤ 1 teaspoon red pepper flakes (optional)

Directions:

1. Remove any leaves from the cauliflower, and cut it into florets.
2. In a large saucepan, bring the water to a boil. Place a steamer basket over the water, and add the florets and salt. Cover and steam for 5 to 7 minutes, until tender.
3. In a large bowl, toss the cauliflower with the red pepper flakes (if using). Transfer the florets to a large airtight container or 6 single-serving containers. Let cool before sealing the lids.

Nutrition: Calories: 35Fat: 0gProtein: 3gCarbohydrates: 7gFiber: 4gSugar: 4gSodium: 236mg

Crusty Grilled Corn

Prep Time:10 minutes

Cook Time:15 minutes

Servings: 4

Ingredients:

- 2 corn cobs
- 1/3 cup Vegenaise
- 1 small handful cilantro
- ½ cup breadcrumbs
- 1 teaspoon lemon juice

Directions:

1. Preheat the gas grill on high heat.
2. Add corn grill to the grill and continue grilling until it turns golden-brown on all sides.
3. Mix the Vegenaise, cilantro, breadcrumbs, and lemon juice in a bowl.
4. Add grilled corn cobs to the crumbs mixture.
5. Toss well then serve.

Nutrition: Calories: 253 Total Fat: 13g Protein: 31g Total Carbs: 3g Fiber: 0g Net Carbs: 3g

Grilled Carrots with Chickpea Salad

Prep Time:10 minutes

Cook Time:10 minutes

Servings: 8

Ingredients:

- ➢ Carrots
- ➢ 8 large carrots
- ➢ 1 tablespoon oil
- ➢ 1 ½ teaspoon salt
- ➢ 1 teaspoon dried oregano
- ➢ 1 teaspoon dried thyme
- ➢ 2 teaspoon paprika powder
- ➢ 1 ½ tablespoon soy sauce
- ➢ ½ cup of water
- ➢ Chickpea Salad
- ➢ 14 oz. canned chickpeas
- ➢ 3 medium pickles
- ➢ 1 small onion
- ➢ A big handful of lettuce
- ➢ 1 teaspoon apple cider vinegar
- ➢ ½ teaspoon dried oregano
- ➢ ½ teaspoon salt
- ➢ Ground black pepper, to taste

➢ ½ cup vegan cream

Directions:

1. Toss the carrots with all of its ingredients in a bowl.
2. Thread one carrot on a stick and place it on a plate.
3. Preheat the grill over high heat.
4. Grill the carrots for 2 minutes per side on the grill.
5. Toss the ingredients for the salad in a large salad bowl.
6. Slice grilled carrots and add them on top of the salad.
7. Serve fresh.

Nutrition: Calories: 661 Total Fat: 68g Carbs: 17g Net Carbs: 7g Fiber: 2g Protein: 4g

Asparagus Spanakopita

Prep Time:25 minutes

Cook Time:25 minutes

Servings: 12

Ingredients:

- ➢ 2 cups cut fresh asparagus (1-inch pieces)
- ➢ 20 sheets phyllo dough, (14 inches x 9 inches)
- ➢ Nonstick cooking spray
- ➢ Refrigerated butter-flavored spray
- ➢ 2 cups torn fresh spinach
- ➢ 3 oz. crumbled feta cheese
- ➢ 2 tablespoon butter
- ➢ 1/4 cup all-purpose flour
- ➢ 1-1/2 cups coconut milk
- ➢ 3 tablespoon lemon juice
- ➢ 1 teaspoon dill weed
- ➢ 1 teaspoon dried thyme
- ➢ 1/4 teaspoon salt

Directions:

1. In a steamer basket, put the asparagus and place it on top of a saucepan with 1-inch of water, then boil. Put the cover and let it steam for 5 minutes or until it becomes crisp-tender.

2. Put 1 sheet of phyllo dough in a cooking spray-coated 13x9-inch baking dish, then cut if needed. Use the butter-flavored spray to spritz the dough. Redo the layers 9 times. Lay the asparagus, feta cheese, and spinach on top. Cover it using a sheet of phyllo dough, then spritz it using the butter-flavored spray. Redo the process using the leftover phyllo. Slice it into 12 pieces. Let it bake for 15 minutes at 350 degrees F without cover, or until it turns golden brown.

3. To make the sauce, in a small saucepan, melt the butter. Mix in the flour until it becomes smooth, then slowly add the milk. Stir in salt, thyme, dill, and lemon juice, then boil. Let it cook and stir for 5 minutes until it becomes thick. Serve the spanakopita with the sauce.

Nutrition: Calories 112 Fat 4 Carbs 14 Protein 5

Black Bean and Corn Salsa from Red Gold

Prep Time:15 minutes

Cook Time:15 minutes

Servings: 25

Ingredients:

- 2 cans black beans, drained and rinsed
- 1 can whole kernel corn, drained
- 2 cans RED GOLD® Petite Diced Tomatoes & Green Chilies
- 1 can RED GOLD® Diced Tomatoes, drained
- 1/2 cup chopped green onions
- 2 tablespoon chopped fresh cilantro
- Salt and black pepper to taste

Directions:

1. Mix all ingredients to combine in a big bowl. Refrigerate to blend flavors for a few hours to overnight. Serve with chips or crackers.

   Nutrition: Calories 65 Fat 3 Carbs 8 Protein 9

Avocado Bean Dip

Prep Time:15 minutes

Cook Time:15 minutes

Servings: 2

Ingredients:

- ➢ 1 medium ripe avocado, peeled and cubed
- ➢ 1/2 cup fresh cilantro leaves
- ➢ 3 tablespoon lime juice
- ➢ 1/2 teaspoon onion powder
- ➢ 1/2 teaspoon garlic powder
- ➢ 1/2 teaspoon chipotle hot pepper sauce
- ➢ 1/4 teaspoon salt
- ➢ 1/4 teaspoon ground cumin
- ➢ Baked tortilla chips

Directions:

1. Mix the first 9 ingredients in a food processor, then cover and blend until smooth. Serve along with chips.

Nutrition: Calories 85 Fat 4 Carbs 13 Protein 6

Crunchy Peanut Butter Apple Dip

Prep Time:10 minutes

Cook Time:10 minutes

Servings: 2

Ingredients:

➢ 1 carton (8 oz.) reduced-fat spreadable cream cheese

➢ 1 cup creamy peanut butter

➢ 1/4 cup coconut milk

➢ 1 tablespoon brown sugar

➢ 1 teaspoon vanilla extract

➢ 1/2 cup chopped unsalted peanuts

➢ Apple slices

Directions:

1. Beat the initial 5 ingredients in a small bowl until combined. Mix in peanuts. Serve with slices of apple, then put the leftovers in the fridge.

Nutrition: Calories 125 Fat 5 Carbs 23 Protein 9

Creamy Cucumber Yogurt Dip

Prep Time:15 minutes

Cook Time:15 minutes

Servings: 4

Ingredients:

- ➤ 1 cup (8 oz.) reduced-fat plain yogurt
- ➤ 4 oz. reduced-fat cream cheese
- ➤ 1/2 cup chopped seeded peeled cucumber
- ➤ 1-1/2 teaspoon. finely chopped onion
- ➤ 1-1/2 teaspoon. snipped fresh dill or 1/2 teaspoon dill weed
- ➤ 1 teaspoon lemon juice
- ➤ 1 teaspoon grated lemon peel
- ➤ 1 garlic clove, minced
- ➤ 1/4 teaspoon salt
- ➤ 1/4 teaspoon pepper
- ➤ Assorted fresh vegetables

Directions:

1. Mix the cream cheese and yogurt in a small bowl. Stir in pepper, salt, garlic, peel, lemon juice, dill, onion, and cucumber. Put on the cover and let it chill in the fridge. Serve it with the veggies.

Nutrition: Calories 55 Fat 4 Carbs 12 Protein 6

Chunky Cucumber Salsa

Prep Time:20 minutes

Cook Time:20 minutes

Servings: 4

Ingredients:

➢ 3 medium cucumbers, peeled and coarsely chopped

➢ 1 medium mango, coarsely chopped

➢ 1 cup frozen corn, thawed

➢ 1 medium sweet red pepper, coarsely chopped

➢ 1 small red onion, coarsely chopped

➢ 1 jalapeno pepper, finely chopped

➢ 3 garlic cloves, minced

➢ 2 tablespoon white wine vinegar

➢ 1 tablespoon minced fresh cilantro

➢ 1 teaspoon salt

➢ 1/2 teaspoon sugar

➢ 1/4 to 1/2 teaspoon cayenne pepper

Directions:

1. Mix all ingredients in a big bowl, then chill, covered, about 2 to 3 hours before serving.

Nutrition: Calories 215 Fat 5 Carbs 23 Protein 10

Steamed Cauliflower

Preparation Time: 5 minutes

Cooking Time: 10 minutes

Servings: 6

Ingredients:

- ➢ 1 large head cauliflower
- ➢ 1 cup water
- ➢ ½ teaspoon salt
- ➢ 1 teaspoon red pepper flakes (optional)

Directions:

1. Remove any leaves from the cauliflower, and cut it into florets.

2. In a large saucepan, bring the water to a boil. Place a steamer basket over the water, and add the florets and salt. Cover and steam for 5 to 7 minutes, until tender.

3. In a large bowl, toss the cauliflower with the red pepper flakes (if using). Transfer the florets to a large airtight container or 6 single-serving containers. Let cool before sealing the lids.

Nutrition: Calories: 35Fat: 0gProtein: 3gCarbohydrates: 7gFiber: 4gSugar: 4gSodium: 236mg

Cajun Sweet Potatoes

Preparation Time: 5 minutes

Cooking Time: 30 minutes

Servings: 4

Ingredients:

- ➢ 2 pounds sweet potatoes
- ➢ 2 teaspoons extra-virgin olive oil
- ➢ ½ teaspoon ground cayenne pepper
- ➢ ½ teaspoon smoked paprika
- ➢ ½ teaspoon dried oregano
- ➢ ½ teaspoon dried thyme
- ➢ ½ teaspoon garlic powder
- ➢ ½ teaspoon salt (optional)

Directions:

1. Preheat the oven to 400ºF. Line a baking sheet with parchment paper.

2. Wash the potatoes, pat dry, and cut into ¾-inch cubes. Transfer to a large bowl, and pour the olive oil over the potatoes.

3. In a small bowl, combine the cayenne, paprika, oregano, thyme, and garlic powder. Sprinkle the spices over the potatoes and combine until the potatoes are well coated. Spread the potatoes on the prepared baking sheet in a single layer. Season

with the salt (if using). Roast for 30 minutes, stirring the potatoes after 15 minutes.

4. Divide the potatoes evenly among 4 single-serving containers. Let cool completely before sealing.

Nutrition: Calories: 219Fat: 3gProtein: 4gCarbohydrates: 46gFiber: 7gSugar: 9gSodium: 125mg

Smoky Coleslaw

Preparation Time: 10 minutes

Cooking Time: 0 minute

Servings: 6

Ingredients:

- ➢ 1-pound shredded cabbage
- ➢ 1/3 cup vegan mayonnaise
- ➢ ¼ cup unseasoned rice vinegar
- ➢ 3 tablespoons plain vegan yogurt or plain soymilk
- ➢ 1 tablespoon vegan sugar
- ➢ ½ teaspoon salt
- ➢ ¼ teaspoon freshly ground black pepper
- ➢ ¼ teaspoon smoked paprika
- ➢ ¼ teaspoon chipotle powder

Directions:

1. Put the shredded cabbage in a large bowl. In a medium bowl, whisk the mayonnaise, vinegar, yogurt, sugar, salt, pepper, paprika, and chipotle powder.

2. Pour over the cabbage, and mix with a spoon or spatula and until the cabbage shreds are coated. Divide the coleslaw evenly among 6 single-serving containers. Seal the lids.

Nutrition: Calories: 73Fat: 4gProtein: 1gCarbohydrates: 8gFiber: 2gSugar: 5gSodium: 283mg

Mediterranean Hummus Pizza

Preparation Time: 10 minutes

Cooking Time: 30 minutes

Servings: 2 pizzas

Ingredients:

- ½ zucchini, thinly sliced
- ½ red onion, thinly sliced
- 1 cup cherry tomatoes, halved
- 2 to 4 tablespoons pitted and chopped black olives
- Pinch sea salt
- Drizzle olive oil (optional)
- 2 prebaked pizza crusts
- ½ cup Classic Hummus
- 2 to 4 tablespoons Cheesy Sprinkle

Directions:

1. Preheat the oven to 400°F. Place the zucchini, onion, cherry tomatoes, and olives in a large bowl, sprinkle them with the sea salt, and toss them a bit. Drizzle with a bit of olive oil (if using), to seal in the flavor and keep them from drying out in the oven.

2. Lay the two crusts out on a large baking sheet. Spread half the hummus on each crust, and top with the veggie mixture and some Cheesy Sprinkle.

Pop the pizzas in the oven for 20 to 30 minutes, or until the veggies are soft.

Nutrition: Calories: 500; Total fat: 25gCarbs: 58gFiber: 12gProtein:

Minted Peas

Preparation Time: 5 minutes

Cooking Time: 5 minutes

Servings: 4

Ingredients:

- ➢ 1 tablespoon olive oil
- ➢ 4 cups peas, fresh or frozen (not canned)
- ➢ ½ teaspoon sea salt
- ➢ freshly ground black pepper
- ➢ 3 tablespoons chopped fresh mint

Directions:

1. In a large sauté pan, heat the olive oil over medium-high heat until hot. Add the peas and cook, about 5 minutes.
2. Remove the pan from heat. Stir in the salt, season with pepper, and stir in the mint.
3. Serve hot.

Nutrition: Calories: 77Fat: 3gProtein: 4gCarbohydrates: 12gFiber: 5gSugar: 3gSodium: 320mg

Glazed Curried Carrots

Preparation Time: 5 minutes

Cooking Time: 15 minutes

Servings: 6

Ingredients:

- ➢ 1-pound carrots, peeled and thinly sliced
- ➢ 2 tablespoons olive oil
- ➢ 2 tablespoons curry powder
- ➢ 2 tablespoons pure maple syrup
- ➢ juice of ½ lemon
- ➢ sea salt
- ➢ freshly ground black pepper

Directions:

1. Place the carrots in a large pot and cover with water. Cook on medium-high heat until tender, about 10 minutes. Drain the carrots and return them to the pan over medium-low heat.

2. Stir in the olive oil, curry powder, maple syrup, and lemon juice. Cook, stirring constantly, until the liquid reduces, about 5 minutes. Season with salt and pepper and serve immediately.

Nutrition: Calories: 171Fat: 3gProtein: 4gCarbohydrates: 34gFiber: 5gSugar: 3gSodium: 129mg

Thai Roasted Broccoli

Preparation Time: 5 minutes

Cooking Time: 15 minutes

Servings: 4

Ingredients:

➢ 1 head broccoli, cut into florets

➢ 2 tablespoons olive oil

➢ 1 tablespoon soy sauce or gluten-free tamari

Directions:

1. Preheat the oven to 425°F. Line a baking sheet with parchment paper. In a large bowl, combine the broccoli, oil, and soy sauce. Toss well to combine.

2. Spread the broccoli on the prepared baking sheet. Roast for 10 minutes.

3. Toss the broccoli with a spatula and roast for an additional 5 minutes, or until the edges of the florets begin to brown.

Nutrition: Calories: 44Fat: 2gProtein: 3gCarbohydrates: 7gFiber: 2gSugar: 3gSodium: 20mg

Coconut Curry Noodle

Preparation Time: 10 minutes

Cooking Time: 30 minutes

Servings: 4

Ingredients:

- ½ tablespoon oil
- 3 garlic cloves, minced
- 2 tablespoons lemongrass, minced
- 1 tablespoon fresh ginger, grated
- 2 tablespoons red curry paste
- 1 (14 oz.) can coconut milk
- 1 tablespoon brown sugar
- 2 tablespoons soy sauce
- 2 tablespoons fresh lime juice
- 1 tablespoon hot chili paste
- 12 oz. linguine
- 2 cups broccoli florets
- 1 cup carrots, shredded
- 1 cup edamame, shelled
- 1 red bell pepper, sliced

Directions:

1. Fill a suitably-sized pot with salted water and boil it on high heat.
2. Add pasta to the boiling water and cook until it is al dente then rinse under cold water.

3. Now place a medium-sized saucepan over medium heat and add oil.
4. Stir in ginger, garlic, and lemongrass, then sauté for 30 seconds.
5. Add coconut milk, soy sauce, curry paste, brown sugar, chili paste, and lime juice.
6. Stir this curry mixture for 10 minutes, or until it thickens.
7. Toss in carrots, broccoli, edamame, bell pepper, and cooked pasta.
8. Mix well, then serve warm.

Nutrition: Calories: 44Fat: 2gProtein: 3gCarbohydrates: 7gFiber: 2gSugar: 3gSodium: 20mg

Collard Green Pasta

Preparation Time: 10 minutes

Cooking Time: 20 minutes

Servings: 4

Ingredients

➢ 2 tablespoons olive oil

➢ 4 garlic cloves, minced

➢ 8 oz. whole wheat pasta

➢ ½ cup panko bread crumbs

➢ 1 tablespoon nutritional yeast

➢ 1 teaspoon red pepper flakes

➢ 1 large bunch collard greens

➢ 1 large lemon, zest and juiced

Directions:

1. Fill a suitable pot with salted water and boil it on high heat.

2. Add pasta to the boiling water and cook until it is al dente, then rinse under cold water.

3. Reserve ½ cup of the cooking liquid from the pasta.

4. Place a non-stick pan over medium heat and add 1 tablespoon olive oil.

5. Stir in half of the garlic, then sauté for 30 seconds.

6. Add breadcrumbs and sauté for approximately 5 minutes.

7. Toss in red pepper flakes and nutritional yeast then mix well.

8. Transfer the breadcrumbs mixture to a plate and clean the pan.

9. Add the remaining tablespoon oil to the nonstick pan.

10. Stir in the garlic clove, salt, black pepper, and chard leaves.

11. Cook for 5 minutes until the leaves are wilted.

12. Add pasta along with the reserved pasta liquid.

13. Mix well, then add garlic crumbs, lemon juice, and zest.

14. Toss well, then serve warm.

Nutrition: Calories: 45Fat: 2.5gProtein: 4gCarbohydrates: 9gFiber: 4gSugar: 3gSodium: 20mg

Glazed Avocado

Preparation Time: 10 minutes

Cooking Time: 12 minutes

Servings: 4

Ingredients:

- ➢ 1 tablespoon stevia
- ➢ 1 teaspoon olive oil
- ➢ 1 teaspoon water
- ➢ 1 teaspoon lemon juice
- ➢ ½ teaspoon rosemary, dried
- ➢ ½ teaspoon ground black pepper
- ➢ 2 avocados, peeled, pitted and cut into large pieces

Directions:

1. Heat up a pan with the oil over medium heat, add the avocados, stevia and the other ingredients, toss, cook for 12 minutes, divide into bowls and serve.

Nutrition: Calories 262 Fat 9.6 Fiber 0.1 Carbs 6.5 Protein 7.9

Mango and Leeks Meatballs

Preparation Time: 20 minutes

Cooking Time: 10 minutes

Servings: 4

Ingredients:

- ➢ 1 tablespoon mango puree
- ➢ 1 cup leeks, chopped
- ➢ ½ cup tofu, crumbled
- ➢ 1 teaspoon dried oregano
- ➢ 1 tablespoon almond flour
- ➢ 1 teaspoon olive oil
- ➢ 1 tablespoon flax meal
- ➢ ½ teaspoon chili flakes

Directions:

1. In the mixing bowl, mix up mango puree with leeks, tofu and the other ingredients except the oil and stir well.
2. Make the small meatballs.
3. After this, pour the olive oil in the skillet and heat it up.
4. Add the meatballs in the skillet and cook them for 4 minutes from each side.

Nutrition: Calories 147 Fat 8.6 Fiber 4.5 Carbs 5.6 Protein 5.3

Spicy Carrots and Olives

Preparation Time: 15 minutes

Cooking Time: 10 minutes

Servings: 4

Ingredients:

➢ ½ teaspoon hot paprika

➢ 1 red chili pepper, minced

➢ ¼ teaspoon ground cumin

➢ ¼ teaspoon dried oregano

➢ ¼ teaspoon dried basil

➢ ½ teaspoon salt

➢ 1 tablespoon olive oil

➢ 1 pound baby carrots, peeled

➢ 1 cup kalamata olives, pitted and halved

➢ juice of 1 lime

Directions:

1. Heat up a pan with the oil over medium heat, add the carrots, olives and the other ingredients, toss, cook for 10 minutes, divide between plates and serve.

Nutrition: Calories 141 Fat 5.8 Fiber 4.3 Carbs 7.5 Protein 9.6

Tamarind Avocado Bowls

Preparation Time: 10 minutes

Cooking Time: 0 minutes

Servings: 2

Ingredients:

- ➢ 1 teaspoon cumin seeds
- ➢ 1 tablespoon olive oil
- ➢ ½ teaspoon gram masala
- ➢ 1 teaspoon ground ginger
- ➢ 2 avocados, peeled, pitted and roughly cubed
- ➢ 1 mango, peeled, and cubed
- ➢ 1 cup cherry tomatoes, halved
- ➢ ½ teaspoon cayenne pepper
- ➢ 1 teaspoon turmeric powder
- ➢ 3 tablespoons tamarind paste

Directions:

1. In a bowl, mix the avocados with the mango and the other ingredients, toss and serve.

Nutrition: Calories 170 Fat 4.5 Fiber 3 Carbs 5 Protein 6

Avocado and Leeks Mix

Preparation Time: 10 minutes

Cooking Time: 0 minutes

Servings: 4

Ingredients:

- ➢ 1 small red onion, chopped
- ➢ 2 avocados, pitted, peeled and chopped
- ➢ 1 teaspoon chili powder
- ➢ 2 leeks, sliced
- ➢ 1 cup cucumber, cubed
- ➢ 1 cup cherry tomatoes, halved
- ➢ Salt and black pepper to the taste
- ➢ 2 tablespoons cumin powder
- ➢ 2 tablespoons lime juice
- ➢ 1 tablespoon parsley, chopped

Directions:

1. In a bowl, mix the onion with the avocados, chili powder and the other ingredients, toss and serve.

Nutrition: Calories 120 Fat 2 Fiber 2 Carbs 7 Protein 4

Cabbage Bowls

Preparation Time: 10 minutes

Cooking Time: 10 minutes

Servings: 4

Ingredients:

- 1 green cabbage head, shredded
- 1 red cabbage head, shredded
- 1 teaspoon garam masala
- 1 teaspoon basil, dried
- 1 teaspoon coriander, ground
- 1 teaspoon mustard seeds
- 1 tablespoon balsamic vinegar
- ¼ cup tomatoes, crushed
- A pinch of salt and black pepper
- 3 carrots, shredded
- 1 yellow bell pepper, chopped
- 1 orange bell pepper, chopped
- 1 red bell pepper, chopped
- 2 tablespoons dill, chopped
- 2 tablespoons olive oil

Directions:

1. Heat up a pan with the oil over medium heat, add the peppers and carrots and cook for 2 minutes.

2. Add the cabbage and the other ingredients, toss, cook for 10 minutes, divide between plates and serve.

Nutrition: Calories 150 Fat 9 Fiber 4 Carbs 3.3 Protein 4.4

Pomegranate and Pears Salad

Preparation Time: 10 minutes

Cooking Time: 0 minutes

Servings: 3

Ingredients:

- ➢ 3 big pears, cored and cut with a spiralizer
- ➢ ¾ cup pomegranate seeds
- ➢ 2 cups baby spinach
- ➢ ½ cup black olives, pitted and cubed
- ➢ ¾ cup walnuts, chopped1 tablespoon olive oil
- ➢ 1 tablespoon coconut sugar
- ➢ 1 teaspoon white sesame seeds
- ➢ 2 tablespoons chives, chopped
- ➢ 1 tablespoon balsamic vinegar
- ➢ 1 garlic clove, minced
- ➢ A pinch of sea salt and black pepper

Directions:

1. In a bowl, mix the pears with the pomegranate seeds, spinach and the other ingredients, toss and serve.

Nutrition: Calories 200 Fat 3.9 Fiber 4 Carbs 6 Protein 3.3

Bulgur and Tomato Mix

Preparation Time: 15 minutes

Cooking Time: 0 minutes

Servings: 4

Ingredients:

- 1 ½ cups hot water
- 1 cup bulgur
- Juice of 1 lime
- 1 cup cherry tomatoes, halved
- 4 tablespoons cilantro, chopped
- ½ cup cranberries, dried
- juice of ½ lemon
- 1 teaspoon oregano, dried
- 1/3 cup almonds, sliced
- ¼ cup green onions, chopped
- ½ cup red bell peppers, chopped
- ½ cup carrots, grated
- 1 tablespoon avocado oil
- A pinch of sea salt and black pepper

Directions:

1. Place bulgur into a bowl, add boiling water to it, stir, and cover and set aside for 15 minutes.
2. Fluff bulgur with a fork and transfer to a bowl.
3. Add the rest of the ingredients, toss and serve.

Nutrition: Calories 260 Fat 4.4 Fiber 3 Carbs 7 Protein 10

Beans Mix

Preparation Time: 10 minutes

Cooking Time: 15 minutes

Servings: 4

Ingredients:

- 1 ½ cups cooked black beans
- 1 cup cooked red kidney beans
- ½ teaspoon garlic powder
- ½ teaspoon smoked paprika
- 2 teaspoons chili powder
- 1 tablespoon olive oil
- 1 ½ cups chickpeas, cooked
- 1 teaspoon garam masala
- 1 red bell pepper, chopped
- 2 tomatoes, chopped
- 1 cup cashews, chopped
- ½ cup veggie stock
- 1 tablespoon balsamic vinegar
- 1 tablespoon oregano, chopped
- 1 tablespoon dill, chopped
- 1 cup corn kernels, chopped

Directions:

1. Heat up a pan with the oil over medium heat, add the beans, garlic powder, chili powder and the other ingredients, toss and cook for 15 minutes.

2. Divide between plates and serve.

Nutrition: Calories 300 Fat 8.3 Fiber 3.3 Carbs 6 Protein 13

Black Bean Burgers

Preparation Time: 10 minutes

Cooking Time: 15 minutes

Servings: 6

Ingredients:

- ➢ 1 Onion, diced
- ➢ ½ cup Corn Nibs
- ➢ 2 Cloves Garlic, minced
- ➢ ½ teaspoon Oregano, dried
- ➢ ½ cup Flour
- ➢ 1 Jalapeno Pepper, small
- ➢ 2 cups Black Beans, mashed & canned
- ➢ ¼ cup Breadcrumbs (Vegan)
- ➢ 2 teaspoons Parsley, minced
- ➢ ¼ teaspoon cumin
- ➢ 1 tablespoon Olive Oil
- ➢ 2 teaspoons Chili Powder
- ➢ ½ Red Pepper, diced
- ➢ Sea Salt to taste

Directions:

1. Set your flour on a plate, and then get out your garlic, onion, peppers and oregano, throwing it in a pan. Cook over medium-high heat, and then cook until the onions are translucent. Place the peppers in, and sauté until tender.

2. Cook for two minutes, and then set it to the side.

3. Use a potato masher to mash your black beans, then stir in the vegetables, cumin, breadcrumbs, parsley, salt, and chili powder, and then divide it into six patties.

4. Coat each side, and then cook until it is fried on each side.

Nutrition: Calories: 357 kcal Protein: 17.93 g Fat: 5.14 g Carbohydrates: 61.64 g

Dijon Maple Burgers

Preparation Time: 20 minutes

Cooking Time: 30 minutes

Servings: 12

Ingredients:

- ➢ 1 Red Bell Pepper
- ➢ 19 ounces Can Chickpeas, rinsed & drained
- ➢ 1 cup Almonds, ground
- ➢ 2 teaspoons Dijon Mustard
- ➢ 1 teaspoon Oregano
- ➢ ½ teaspoon Sage
- ➢ 1 cup Spinach, fresh
- ➢ 1 – ½ cups Rolled Oats
- ➢ 1 Clove Garlic, pressed
- ➢ ½ Lemon, juiced
- ➢ 2 teaspoons Maple Syrup, pure

Directions:

1. Get out a baking sheet. Line it with parchment paper.

2. Cut your red pepper in half and then take the seeds out. Place it on your baking sheet, and roast in the oven while you prepare your other ingredients.

3. Process your chickpeas, almonds, mustard, and maple syrup together in a food processor.

4. Add in your lemon juice, oregano, sage, garlic, and spinach, processing again. Make sure it's combined, but don't puree it.

5. Once your red bell pepper is softened, which should roughly take ten minutes, add this to the processor as well. Add in your oats, mixing well.

6. Form twelve patties, cooking in the oven for a half-hour. They should be browned.

Nutrition: Calories: 96 kcal Protein: 5.28 g Fat: 2.42 g Carbohydrates: 16.82 g

Hearty Black Lentil Curry

Preparation Time: 30 minutes

Cooking Time: 6 hours and 15 minutes

Servings: 4

Ingredients:

- ➢ 1 cup of black lentils, rinsed and soaked overnight
- ➢ 14 ounce of chopped tomatoes
- ➢ 2 large white onions, peeled and sliced
- ➢ 1 1/2 teaspoon of minced garlic
- ➢ 1 teaspoon of grated ginger
- ➢ 1 red chili
- ➢ 1 teaspoon of salt
- ➢ 1/4 teaspoon of red chili powder
- ➢ 1 teaspoon of paprika
- ➢ 1 teaspoon of ground turmeric
- ➢ 2 teaspoons of ground cumin
- ➢ 2 teaspoons of ground coriander
- ➢ 1/2 cup of chopped coriander
- ➢ 4-ounce of vegetarian butter
- ➢ 4 fluid of ounce water
- ➢ 2 fluid of ounce vegetarian double cream

Directions:

1. Place a large pan over moderate heat, add butter and let heat until melt.

2. Add the onion and garlic and ginger and cook for 10 to 15 minutes or until onions are caramelized.
3. Then stir in salt, red chili powder, paprika, turmeric, cumin, ground coriander, and water.
4. Transfer this mixture to a 6-quarts slow cooker and add tomatoes and red chili.
5. Drain lentils, add to slow cooker, and stir until just mix.
6. Plugin slow cooker; adjust cooking time to 6 hours and let cook on low heat setting.
7. When the lentils are done, stir in cream and adjust the seasoning.
8. Serve with boiled rice or whole wheat bread.

Nutrition: Calories: 299 kcal Protein: 5.59 g Fat: 27.92 g Carbohydrates: 9.83 g

Flavorful Refried Beans

Preparation Time: 15 minutes

Cooking Time: 8 hours

Servings: 8

Ingredients:

- ➢ 3 cups of pinto beans, rinsed
- ➢ 1 small jalapeno pepper, seeded and chopped
- ➢ 1 medium-sized white onion, peeled and sliced
- ➢ 2 tablespoons of minced garlic
- ➢ 5 teaspoons of salt
- ➢ 2 teaspoons of ground black pepper
- ➢ 1/4 teaspoon of ground cumin
- ➢ 9 cups of water

Directions:

1. Using a 6-quarts slow cooker, place all the ingredients and stir until it mixes properly.
2. Cover the top, plug in the slow cooker, adjust the cooking time to 6 hours, let it cook on the high heat setting, and add more water if the beans get too dry.
3. When the beans are done, drain it then reserve the liquid.
4. Mash the beans using a potato masher and pour in the reserved cooking liquid until it reaches your desired mixture.

5. Serve immediately.

Nutrition: Calories: 268 kcal Protein: 16.55 g Fat: 1.7 g Carbohydrates: 46.68 g

Smoky Red Beans and Rice

Preparation Time: 15 minutes

Cooking Time: 6 minutes

Servings: 6

Ingredients:

➢ 30 ounce of cooked red beans

➢ 1 cup of brown rice, uncooked

➢ 1 cup of chopped green pepper

➢ 1 cup of chopped celery

➢ 1 cup of chopped white onion

➢ 1 1/2 teaspoon of minced garlic

➢ 1/2 teaspoon of salt

➢ 1/4 teaspoon of cayenne pepper

➢ 1 teaspoon of smoked paprika

➢ 2 teaspoons of dried thyme

➢ 1 bay leaf

➢ 2 1/3 cups of vegetable broth

Directions:

1. Using a 6-quarts slow cooker, place all the ingredients except for the rice, salt, and cayenne pepper.

2. Stir until it mixes properly and then cover the top.

3. Plug in the slow cooker, adjust the cooking time to 4 hours, and steam on a low heat setting.

4. Then pour in and stir the rice, salt, cayenne pepper and continue cooking for an additional 2 hours at a high heat setting.

5. Serve straight away.

Nutrition: Calories: 791 kcal Protein: 3.25 g Fat: 86.45 g Carbohydrates: 9.67 g

Creamy Artichoke Soup

Preparation Time: 5 minutes

Cooking Time: 40 minutes

Servings: 4

Ingredients:

- ➢ 1 can artichoke hearts, drained
- ➢ 3 cups vegetable broth
- ➢ 2 tbsp. lemon juice
- ➢ 1 small onion, finely cut
- ➢ 2 cloves garlic, crushed
- ➢ 3 tbsp. olive oil
- ➢ 2 tbsp. flour
- ➢ ½ cup vegan cream

Directions:

1. Gently sauté the onion and garlic in some olive oil. Add the flour, whisking constantly, and then add the hot vegetable broth slowly, while still whisking. Cook for about 5 minutes.

2. Blend the artichoke, lemon juice, salt, and pepper until smooth. Add the puree to the broth mix, stir well, and then stir in the cream. Cook until heated through. Garnish with a swirl of vegan cream or a sliver of artichoke.

Nutrition: Calories: 1622 kcal Protein: 4.45 g Fat: 181.08 g Carbohydrates: 10.99 g

Beauty School Ginger Cucumbers

Preparation Time: 10 minutes

Cooking Time: 45 minutes

Servings: 14

Ingredients:

➢ 1 sliced cucumber

➢ 3 tsp. rice wine vinegar

➢ 1 ½ tbsp. sugar

➢ 1 tsp. minced ginger

Directions:

1. Place all together the ingredients in a mixing bowl, and toss the ingredients well. Enjoy!

Nutrition: Calories: 10 kcal Protein: 0.46 g Fat: 0.43 g Carbohydrates: 0.89 g

Sage Walnuts and Radishes

Preparation Time: 10 minutes

Cooking Time: 10 minutes

Servings: 6

Ingredients:

- 2 tablespoons olive oil
- 5 celery ribs, chopped
- 3 spring onions, chopped
- ½ pound radishes, halved
- juice of 1 lime
- Zest of 1 lime, grated
- 8 ounces walnuts, chopped
- A pinch of black pepper
- 3 tablespoons sage, chopped

Directions:

1. Heat up a pan with the oil over medium heat, add celery and spring onion, stir and cook for 5 minutes.

2. Add the rest of the ingredients, toss, cook for another 5 minutes, divide into bowls and serve.

Nutrition: Calories 200 Fat 7 Fiber 5 Carbs 9.3 Protein 4

Crusty Grilled Corn

Preparation Time: 10 minutes

Cooking Time: 15 minutes

Servings: 4

Ingredients:

- ➢ 2 corn cobs
- ➢ 1/3 cup Vegenaise
- ➢ 1 small handful cilantro
- ➢ ½ cup breadcrumbs
- ➢ 1 teaspoon lemon juice

Directions:

6. Preheat the gas grill on high heat.

7. Add corn grill to the grill and continue grilling until it turns golden-brown on all sides.

8. Mix the Vegenaise, cilantro, breadcrumbs, and lemon juice in a bowl.

9. Add grilled corn cobs to the crumbs mixture.

10. Toss well then serve.

Nutrition: Calories: 253 Total Fat: 13g Protein: 31g Total Carbs: 3g Fiber: 0g Net Carbs: 3g

Grilled Carrots with Chickpea Salad

Preparation Time: 10 minutes

Cooking Time: 10 minutes

Servings: 8

Ingredients:

➢ Carrots

➢ 8 large carrots

➢ 1 tablespoon oil

➢ 1 ½ teaspoon salt

➢ 1 teaspoon dried oregano

➢ 1 teaspoon dried thyme

➢ 2 teaspoon paprika powder

➢ 1 ½ tablespoon soy sauce

➢ ½ cup of water

➢ Chickpea Salad

➢ 14 oz. canned chickpeas

➢ 3 medium pickles

➢ 1 small onion

➢ A big handful of lettuce

➢ 1 teaspoon apple cider vinegar

➢ ½ teaspoon dried oregano

➢ ½ teaspoon salt

➢ Ground black pepper, to taste

➢ ½ cup vegan cream

Directions:

8. Toss the carrots with all of its ingredients in a bowl.

9. Thread one carrot on a stick and place it on a plate.

10. Preheat the grill over high heat.

11. Grill the carrots for 2 minutes per side on the grill.

12. Toss the ingredients for the salad in a large salad bowl.

13. Slice grilled carrots and add them on top of the salad.

14. Serve fresh.

Nutrition: Calories: 661 Total Fat: 68g Carbs: 17g Net Carbs: 7g Fiber: 2g Protein: 4g

Grilled Avocado Guacamole

Preparation Time: 10 minutes

Cooking Time: 20 minutes

Servings: 4

Ingredients:

- ½ teaspoon olive oil
- 1 lime, halved
- ½ onion, halved
- 1 serrano chile, halved, stemmed, and seeded
- 3 Haas avocados, skin on
- 2–3 tablespoons fresh cilantro, chopped
- ½ teaspoon smoked salt

Directions:

1. Preheat the grill over medium heat.
2. Brush the grilling grates with olive oil and place chile, onion, and lime on it.
3. Grill the onion for 10 minutes, chile for 5 minutes, and lime for 2 minutes.
4. Transfer the veggies to a large bowl.
5. Now cut the avocados in half and grill them for 5 minutes.
6. Mash the flesh of the grilled avocado in a bowl.
7. Chop the other grilled veggies and add them to the avocado mash.
8. Stir in remaining ingredients and mix well.

9. Serve.

Nutrition: Calories: 165 Total Fat: 17g Carbs: 4g Net Carbs: 2g Fiber: 1g Protein: 1g

Tofu Hoagie Rolls

Preparation Time: 10 minutes

Cooking Time: 20 minutes

Servings: 6

Ingredients:

➢ ½ cup vegetable broth

➢ ¼ cup hot sauce

➢ 1 tablespoon vegan butter

➢ 1 (16 ounce) package tofu, pressed and diced

➢ 4 cups cabbage, shredded

➢ 2 medium apples, grated

➢ 1 medium shallot, grated

➢ 6 tablespoons vegan mayonnaise

➢ 1 tablespoon apple cider vinegar

➢ Salt and black pepper

➢ 4 6-inch hoagie rolls, toasted

Directions:

1. In a saucepan, combine broth with butter and hot sauce and bring to a boil.

2. Add tofu and reduce the heat to a simmer.

3. Cook for 10 minutes then remove from heat and let sit for 10 minutes to marinate.

4. Toss cabbage and rest of the ingredients in a salad bowl.

5. Prepare and set up a grill on medium heat.

6. Drain the tofu and grill for 5 minutes per side.

7. Lay out the toasted hoagie rolls and add grilled tofu to each hoagie

8. Add the cabbage mixture evenly between them then close it.

9. Serve.

Nutrition: Calories: 111 Total Fat: 11g Carbs: 5g Net Carbs: 1g Fiber: 0g Protein: 1g

Grilled Seitan with Creole Sauce

Preparation Time: 10 minutes

Cooking Time: 14 minutes

Servings: 4

Ingredients:

Grilled Seitan Kebabs:

➢ 4 cups seitan, diced

➢ 2 medium onions, diced into squares

➢ 8 bamboo skewers

➢ 1 can coconut milk

➢ 2½ tablespoons creole spice

➢ 2 tablespoons tomato paste

➢ 2 cloves of garlic

Creole Spice Mix:

➢ 2 tablespoons paprika

➢ 12 dried peri chili peppers

➢ 1 tablespoon salt

➢ 1 tablespoon freshly ground pepper

➢ 2 teaspoons dried thyme

➢ 2 teaspoons dried oregano

Directions:

1. Prepare the creole seasoning by blending all its ingredients and preserve in a sealable jar.

2. Thread seitan and onion on the bamboo skewers in an alternating pattern.

3. On a baking sheet, mix coconut milk with creole seasoning, tomato paste and garlic.

4. Soak the skewers in the milk marinade for 2 hours.

5. Prepare and set up a grill over medium heat.

6. Grill the skewers for 7 minutes per side.

7. Serve.

Nutrition: Calories: 407 Total Fat: 42g Carbs: 13g Net Carbs: 6g Fiber: 1g Protein: 4g

Mushroom Steaks

Preparation Time: 10 minutes

Cooking Time: 24 minutes

Servings: 4

Ingredients:

➢ 1 tablespoon vegan butter

➢ ½ cup vegetable broth

➢ ½ small yellow onion, diced

➢ 1 large garlic clove, minced

➢ 3 tablespoons balsamic vinegar

➢ 1 tablespoon mirin

➢ ½ tablespoon soy sauce

➢ ½ tablespoon tomato paste

➢ 1 teaspoon dried thyme

➢ ½ teaspoon dried basil

➢ A dash of ground black pepper

➢ 2 large, whole portobello mushrooms

Directions:

1. Melt butter in a saucepan over medium heat and stir in half of the broth.

2. Bring to a simmer then add garlic and onion. Cook for 8 minutes.

3. Whisk the rest of the ingredients except the mushrooms in a bowl.

4. Add this mixture to the onion in the pan and mix well.
5. Bring this filling to a simmer then remove from the heat.
6. Clean the mushroom caps inside and out and divide the filling between the mushrooms.
7. Place the mushrooms on a baking sheet and top them with remaining sauce and broth.
8. Cover with foil then place it on a grill to smoke.
9. Cover the grill and broil for 16 minutes over indirect heat.
10. Serve warm.

Nutrition: Calories: 887 Total Fat: 93g Carbs: 29g Net Carbs: 13g Fiber: 4g Protein: 8g

Grilled Portobello

Preparation Time: 10 minutes

Cooking Time: 8 minutes

Servings: 04

Ingredients:

- ➢ 4 portobello mushrooms
- ➢ ¼ cup soy sauce
- ➢ ¼ cup tomato sauce
- ➢ 2 tablespoons maple syrup
- ➢ 1 tablespoon molasses
- ➢ 2 tablespoons minced garlic
- ➢ 1 tablespoon onion powder
- ➢ 1 pinch salt and pepper

Directions:

1. Mix all the ingredients except mushrooms in a bowl.
2. Add mushrooms to this marinade and mix well to coat.
3. Cover and marinate for 1 hour.
4. Prepare and set up the grill at medium heat. Grease it with cooking spray.
5. Grill the mushroom for 4 minutes per side.
6. Serve

Nutrition: Calories: 404 Total Fat: 43g Carbs: 8g Net Carbs: 4g Fiber: 1g Protein: 4g

Wok Fried Broccoli

Preparation Time: 10 minutes

Cooking Time: 16 minutes

Servings: 02

Ingredients:

- ➤ 3 ounces whole, blanched peanuts
- ➤ 2 tablespoons olive oil
- ➤ 1 banana shallot, sliced
- ➤ 10 ounces broccoli, trimmed and cut into florets
- ➤ ¼ red pepper, julienned
- ➤ ½ yellow pepper, julienned
- ➤ 1 teaspoon soy sauce

Directions:

1. Toast peanuts on a baking sheet for 15 minutes at 350 degrees F.
2. In a wok, add oil and shallots and sauté for 10 minutes.
3. Toss in broccoli and peppers.
4. Stir fry for 3 minutes then add the rest of the ingredients.
5. Cook for 3 additional minutes and serve.

Nutrition: Calories: 391 Total Fat: 39g Carbs: 15g Net Carbs: 5g Fiber: 2g Protein: 6g

Broccoli & Brown Rice Satay

Preparation Time: 10 minutes

Cooking Time: 10 minutes

Servings: 4

Ingredients:

- 6 trimmed broccoli florets, halved
- 1-inch piece of ginger, shredded
- 2 garlic cloves, shredded
- 1 red onion, sliced
- 1 roasted red pepper, cut into cubes
- 2 teaspoons olive oil
- 1 teaspoon mild chili powder
- 1 tablespoon reduced salt soy sauce
- 1 tablespoon maple syrup
- 1 cup cooked brown rice

Directions:

1. Boil broccoli in water for 4 minutes then drain immediately.
2. In a pan add olive oil, ginger, onion, and garlic.
3. Stir fry for 2 minutes then add the rest of the ingredients.
4. Cook for 3 minutes then serve.

Nutrition: Calories: 196 Total Fat: 20g Carbs: 8g Net Carbs: 3g Fiber: 1g Protein: 3g

Sautéed Sesame Spinach

Preparation Time: 1 hr. 10 minutes

Cooking Time: 3 minutes

Servings: 04

Ingredients:

- 1 tablespoon toasted sesame oil
- ½ tablespoon soy sauce
- ½ teaspoon toasted sesame seeds, crushed
- ½ teaspoon rice vinegar
- ½ teaspoon golden caster sugar
- 1 garlic clove, grated
- 8 ounces spinach, stem ends trimmed

Directions:

1. Sauté spinach in a pan until it is wilted.
2. Whisk the sesame oil, garlic, sugar, vinegar, sesame seeds, soy sauce and black pepper together in a bowl.
3. Stir in spinach and mix well.
4. Cover and refrigerate for 1 hour.
5. Serve.

Nutrition: Calories: 677 Total Fat: 60g Carbs: 71g Net Carbs: 7g Fiber: 0g; Protein: 20g

Fry Noodles

Preparation Time: 10 minutes

Cooking Time: 8 minutes

Servings: 4

Ingredients:

- ➢ 1 cup broccoli, chopped
- ➢ 1 cup red bell pepper, chopped
- ➢ 1 cup mushrooms, chopped
- ➢ 1 large onion, chopped
- ➢ 1 batch Stir Fry Sauce, prepared
- ➢ Salt and black pepper, to taste
- ➢ 2 cups spaghetti, cooked
- ➢ 4 garlic cloves, minced
- ➢ 2 tablespoons sesame oil

Directions:

1. Heat sesame oil in a pan over medium heat and add garlic, onions, bell pepper, broccoli, mushrooms.
2. Sauté for about 5 minutes and add spaghetti noodles and stir fry sauce.
3. Mix well and cook for 3 more minutes.
4. Dish out in plates and serve to enjoy.

Nutrition: Calories: 567 Total fat: 48g Total carbs: 6g Fiber: 4g; Net carbs: 2g Sodium: 373mg Protein: 33g

Spicy Sweet Chili Veggie Noodles

Preparation Time: 10 minutes

Cooking Time: 7 minutes

Servings: 2

Ingredients:

- ➢ 1 head of broccoli, cut into bite sized florets
- ➢ 1 onion, finely sliced
- ➢ 1 tablespoon olive oil
- ➢ 1 courgette, halved
- ➢ 2 nests of whole-wheat noodles
- ➢ 150g mushrooms, sliced
- ➢ For Sauce
- ➢ 3 tablespoons soy sauce
- ➢ ¼ cup sweet chili sauce
- ➢ 1 teaspoon Sriracha
- ➢ 1 tablespoon peanut butter
- ➢ 2 tablespoons boiled water
- ➢ For Topping
- ➢ 2 teaspoons sesame seeds
- ➢ 2 teaspoons dried chili flakes

Directions:

1. Heat olive oil on medium heat in a saucepan and add onions.

2. Sauté for about 2 minutes and add broccoli, courgette and mushrooms.

3. Cook for about 5 minutes, stirring occasionally.

4. Whisk sweet chili sauce, soy sauce, Sriracha, water and peanut butter in a bowl.

5. Cook the noodles according to packet instructions and add to the vegetables.

6. Stir in the sauce and top with dried chili flakes and sesame seeds to serve.

Nutrition: Calories: 351 Total Fat: 27g Protein: 25g Total Carbs: 2g Fiber: 1g Net Carbs: 1g

Creamy Vegan Mushroom Pasta

Preparation Time: 10 minutes

Cooking Time: 30 minutes

Servings: 6

Ingredients:

➢ 2 cups frozen peas, thawed

➢ 3 tablespoons flour, unbleached

➢ 3 cups almond breeze, unsweetened

➢ 1 tablespoon nutritional yeast

➢ 1/3 cup fresh parsley, chopped, plus extra for garnish

➢ ¼ cup olive oil

➢ 1 pound pasta of choice

➢ 4 cloves garlic, minced

➢ 2/3 cup shallots, chopped

➢ 8 cups mixed mushrooms, sliced

➢ Salt and black pepper, to taste

Directions:

1. Take a bowl and boil pasta in salted water.

2. Heat olive oil in a pan over medium heat.

3. Add mushrooms, garlic, shallots and ½ tsp salt and cook for 15 minutes.

4. Sprinkle flour on the vegetables and stir for a minute while cooking.

5. Add almond beverage, stir constantly.

6. Let it simmer for 5 minutes and add pepper to it.

7. Cook for 3 more minutes and remove from heat.

8. Stir in nutritional yeast.

9. Add peas, salt, and pepper.

10. Cook for another minute and add

11. Add pasta to this sauce.

12. Garnish and serve!

Nutrition: Calories: 364 Total Fat: 28g Protein: 24g Total Carbs: 4g Fiber: 2g Net Carbs: 2g

Vegetable Penne Pasta

Preparation Time: 15 minutes

Cooking Time: 20 minutes

Servings: 6

Ingredients:

- ½ large onion, chopped
- 2 celery sticks, chopped
- ½ tablespoon ginger paste
- ½ cup green bell pepper
- 1½ tablespoons soy sauce
- ½ teaspoon parsley
- Salt and black pepper, to taste
- ½ pound penne pasta, cooked
- 2 large carrots, diced
- ½ small leek, chopped
- 1 tablespoon olive oil
- ½ teaspoon garlic paste
- ½ tablespoon Worcester sauce
- ½ teaspoon coriander
- 1 cup water

Directions:

1. Heat olive oil in a wok on medium heat and add onions, garlic and ginger paste.
2. Sauté for about 3 minutes and stir in all bell pepper, celery sticks, carrots and leek.

3. Sauté for about 5 minutes and add remaining ingredients except for pasta.

4. Cover the lid and cook for about 12 minutes.

5. Stir in the cooked pasta and dish out to serve warm.

Nutrition: Calories: 385 Total Fat: 29g Protein: 26g Total Carbs: 5g Fiber: 1g Net Carbs: 4g

Creamy Vegan Spinach Pasta

Preparation Time: 20 minutes

Cooking Time: 5 minutes

Servings: 4

Ingredients:

- ➢ 1 cup raw cashews, soaked in water for 8 hours
- ➢ 2 tablespoons lemon juice
- ➢ 1 tablespoon olive oil
- ➢ 1½ cups vegetable broth
- ➢ 2 tablespoons fresh dill, chopped
- ➢ Red pepper flakes, to taste
- ➢ 10 ounces dried fusilli
- ➢ ½ cup almond milk, unflavored and unsweetened
- ➢ 2 tablespoons white miso paste
- ➢ 4 garlic cloves, divided
- ➢ 8-ounces fresh spinach, finely chopped
- ➢ ¼ cup scallions, chopped
- ➢ Salt and black pepper, to taste

Directions:

1. Boil salted water in a large pot and add pasta.
2. Cook according to the package directions and drain the pasta into a colander.
3. Dish out the pasta in a large serving bowl and add a dash of olive oil to prevent sticking.

4. Put the cashews, milk, miso, lemon juice, and 1 garlic clove into the food processor and blend until smooth.

5. Put olive oil over medium heat in a large pot and add the remaining 3 cloves of garlic.

6. Sauté for about 1 minute and stir in the spinach and broth.

7. Raise the heat and allow to simmer for about 4 minutes until the spinach is bright green and wilted.

8. Stir in the pasta and cashew mixture and season with salt and black pepper.

9. Top with scallions and dill and dish out into plates to serve.

Nutrition: Calories: 94 Total Fat: 10g Protein: 0g Total Carbs: 1g Fiber: 0.3g Net Carbs: 0.7g

Pinto Bean Stew with Cauliflower

Preparation Time: 10 min

Cooking Time: 25 min

Servings: 2

Ingredients:

- 1 cup water
- 1 teaspoon salt
- ¼ cup pinto beans
- 2 tablespoons coconut oil
- ½ small onion chopped
- 1 small zucchini chopped
- ½ teaspoon garlic powder
- 1 bay leaf
- 1 1/2 cups low sodium vegetable stock
- ½ cup steamed cauliflower
- ¼ cup grated mozzarella
- 1 tablespoon chopped fresh cilantro

Directions:

1. In a large bowl, dissolve 1 tablespoon of salt in the water. Add the pinto beans and soak at room temperature for 8 to 24 hours. Drain and rinse.

2. Select Sauté and adjust to Normal or Medium heat. Add the coconut oil to the Instant Pot and heat until shimmering. Add the onion and zucchini, and sprinkle with salt. Cook, stirring often, until the

onion pieces separate and soften. Add the garlic powder and cook for about 1 minute, or until fragrant. Add the drained pinto beans, remaining ¼ teaspoon of salt, bay leaf, and vegetable stock.

3. Lock the lid into place. Select Pressure Cook or Manual, and adjust the pressure to High and the time to 15 minutes. After cooking, let the pressure release naturally for 10 minutes, then quick release any remaining pressure.

4. Unlock the lid. Stir in the cauliflower and bring to a simmer to heat it through and thicken the sauce slightly. Taste the beans and adjust the seasoning. Ladle into bowls and sprinkle with the mozzarella cheese and cilantro.

Nutrition: Calories 245, Total Fat 16. 2g, Saturated Fat 13. 7g, Cholesterol 2mg, Sodium 1745mg, Total Carbohydrate 22. 4g , Dietary Fiber 5.6g , Total Sugars 4. 5g, Protein 7.7g

Tempeh White Bean Gravy

Preparation Time: 05 min

Cooking Time: 20 min

Servings: 2

Ingredients:

- ½ cup cups vegetable broth
- ¼ cup soy sauce
- ¼ cup coconut oil
- 1 teaspoon garlic powder
- ½ cup chopped onion
- 1 cup chopped tempeh
- 1/8 teaspoon dried basil
- 1/8 teaspoon dried parsley
- 1/8 teaspoon ground black pepper
- 1 cup white beans, drained and rinsed
- Enough water

Directions:

1. Add vegetable broth, soy sauce, coconut oil, garlic powder, onion, tempeh, basil, parsley, black pepper and white beans to the Instant Pot. Pour the remaining ¼ cup water over everything.
2. Choose the soup function for 20 minutes.
3. Once done, remove the lid.
4. Serve and enjoy.

Nutrition: Calories 376, Total Fat 29. 4g, Saturated Fat 23. 6g, Cholesterol 0mg, Sodium 2233mg, Total Carbohydrate 22. 4g, Dietary Fiber 4. 9g, Total Sugars 4. 2g, Protein 9. 2g

Broccoli and Black Bean Chili

Preparation Time: 15 min

Cooking Time: 15 min

Servings: 2

Ingredients:

➢ ½ tablespoon coconut oil

➢ 1 cup broccoli

➢ 1 cup chopped red onions

➢ ½ tablespoon paprika

➢ 1/2 teaspoon salt

➢ ¼ cup tomatoes

➢ 1 cup black beans drained, rinsed

➢ ¼ chopped green chills

➢ ½ cup water

Directions:

1. In the Instant Pot, select Sauté; adjust to normal. Heat coconut oil in Instant Pot. Add broccoli, onions, paprika and salt; cook 8 to 10 minutes, stirring occasionally, until thoroughly cooked. Select Cancel.

2. Stir in tomatoes, black beans, chills and water. Secure lid, set pressure valve to Sealing. Select manual, cook on High pressure 5 minutes. Select Cancel. Keep pressure valve in sealing position to release pressure naturally.

Nutrition: Calories 408, Total Fat 5. 3g, Saturated Fat 3. 4g, Cholesterol 0mg, Sodium 607mg, Total Carbohydrate 70. 7g, Dietary Fiber 18. 1g, Total Sugars 6g, Protein 23. 3g